Chemo Cupcakes and Carpools

Keeping Your Gratitude Intact

JOURNAL

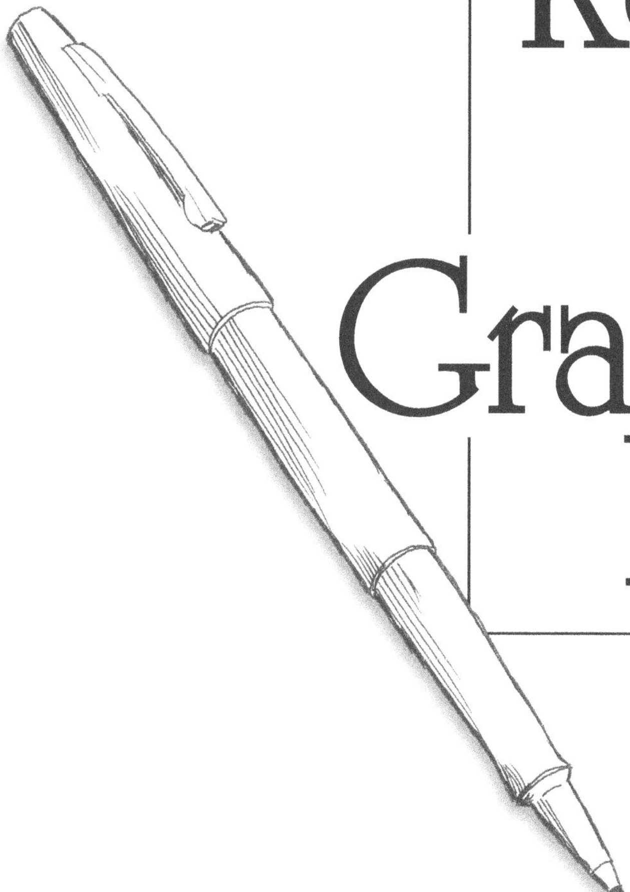

ANGELIQUE L'AMOUR

Chemo, Cupcakes and Carpool
Keeping Your Gratitude Intact
Journal

ISBN: 978-0-9975444-3-5

Angelique L'Amour
Angelique L'Amour Pitney, Pub
Published by Angelique L'Amour Pitney, Publishing
Los Angeles, CA

Dedication

To My Fellow Survivors — You are the reason I did this!

Gratitude

Welcome to the companion to *Chemo, Cupcakes and Carpools*.
I created this gratitude journal based off of my own journal entries.
This is meant to be written in and explored.

A number of studies prove that finding the gratitude in each day changes your point of view. You will find yourself to be calmer and more appreciative of the life you have. While this can be a challenge during a time of great stress, it can also be a lifesaver. Hopefully what follows will bring a smile, a chuckle, a dream, and some hope.

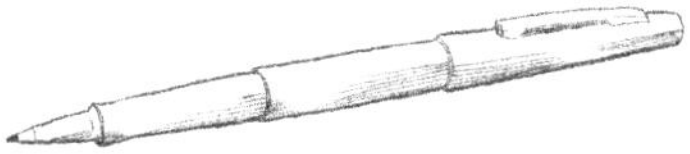

Gratitude Page

Take a moment as often as you can to write down something you are grateful for from lip balm to your children to ice cream. Ask your kids to do it too—it changes your day instantly.

Journal

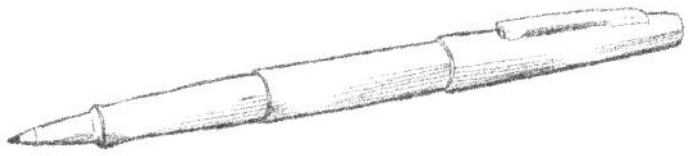

People I have met

List people you have met that are now invaluable and that you never would have met without a cancer diagnosis. I have several new friends that are a constant part of my life and I am so grateful to have them.

Journal

Where do you want to travel?

Countries
(for me it's Greece)

Hotels you want to stay at

Restaurants you want
to eat at

Journal

List the things that make you happy

Seeing a sunrise, taking a walk, petting your dog — Plan to do one of them asap!

To See	To Do	To Feel

Journal

What do you believe about faith?

Journal

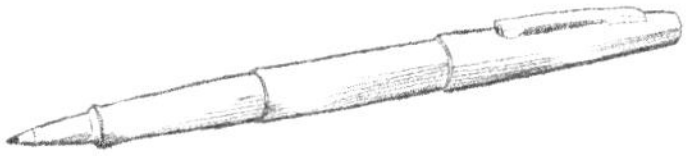

What do you want to learn?

I have always wanted to learn French!

Journal

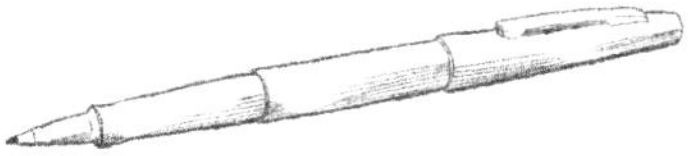

What do you want your kids to learn?

...by seeing how you handle these challenges.

Journal

What do you want to buy?

...warm socks, a new slow cooker.

Journal

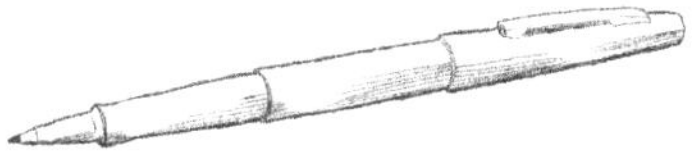

What do you want to improve?

Patience? Cooking?

Journal

What do you like to eat?

Journal

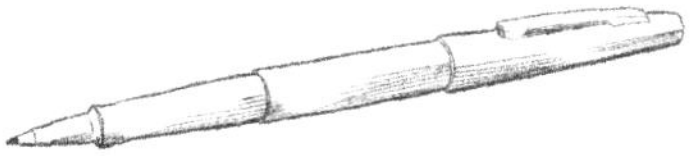

What recipes do you like?

Journal

Who do you appreciate in your life?

The valet parkers at my oncologist were amazing and kind.

Journal

What are you not telling anyone?

Journal

What do you want to feel?

Brave? Strong? Hopeful? Happy?

Journal

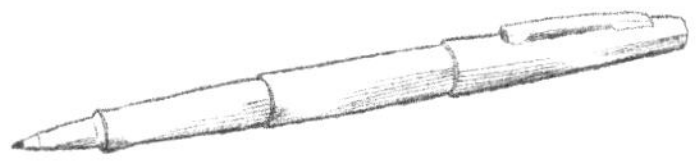

What do you need to do to feel that way?

List some steps that will make this happen.

Journal

What do you need to organize?

Journal

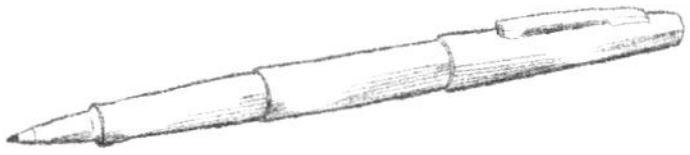

What do you want to make?

Journal

What makes your spouse happy that you can do right now?

Journal

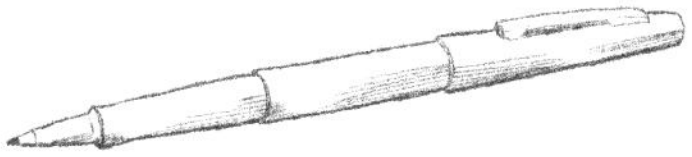

What makes each of your kids happy that you can do right now?

We went for muffins at a bakery on the way to school on late start Wednesday.

Journal

Holiday gift list

Journal

Birthdays to remember

Website: angeliquelamour.com

Book: angeliquelamour.com/books/chemo-cupcakes-and-carpools/

Twitter: @LAmourAngelique

Facebook: www.facebook.com/angeliquelamourauthor

Instagram: www.instagram.com/angeliquelamourauthor/

Goodreads: Angelique L'Amour

Biography

Angelique L'Amour was born in Los Angeles, California. The daughter of author Louis L'Amour, she grew up in the household of a prolific writer where writing and storytelling were a way of life. In 1988, Angelique created and edited a volume of quotes from her father's works. Published by Bantam Doubleday Dell in 1988, *A Trail of Memories* spent 16 weeks on the *New York Times* bestseller list and was also a *Publisher's Weekly* bestseller for 1988. Angelique has spent the past 20 years as a freelance editor working on academic paper, novels and film projects as well as writing content for two websites. She also created and taught a Creative Writing program for students from 8 to 80 and is contemplating developing that into an online and book course. Future projects include a spiritual self-help book as well as several novels. A wife, mother of two and a breast cancer survivor, time is also spent promoting early detection by teaching, speaking engagements and writing her blog, *My Story Right Now* which can be found through her website: angeliquelamour.com
Her current book, *Chemo, Cupcakes and Carpools* is available now wherever books are sold.

Made in the USA
Monee, IL
05 November 2026

67375708R00031